BABY SIGN LANGUAGE BOOK

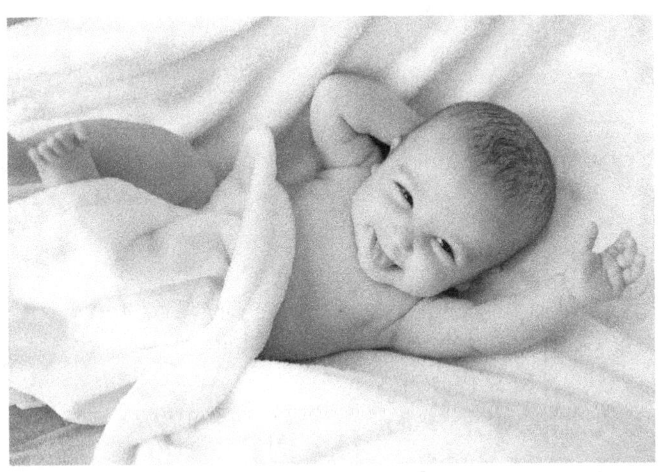

50 Priority Signs And Easy Ways To Start Communicating With Your Child

HUNTER MOODY

TABLE OF CONTENTS

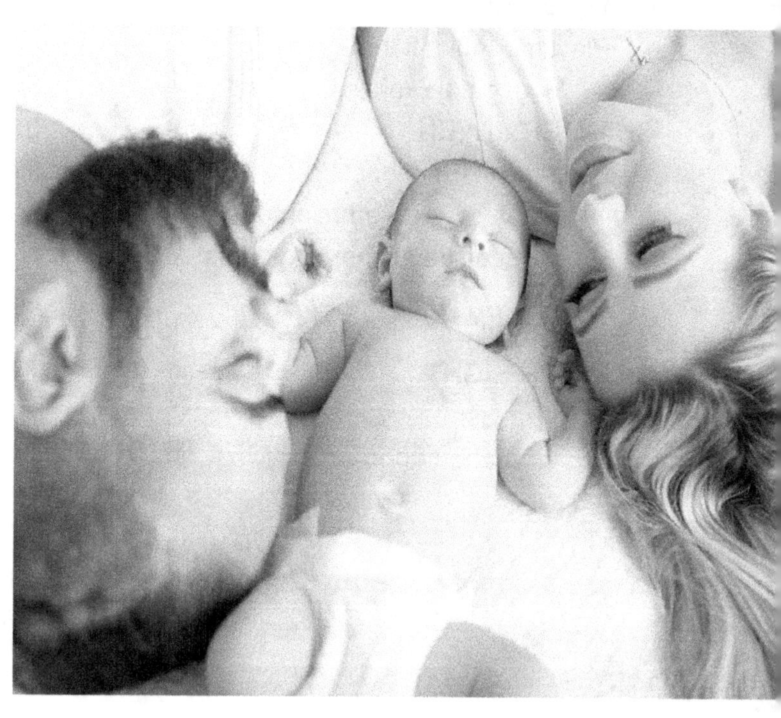

INTRODUCTION

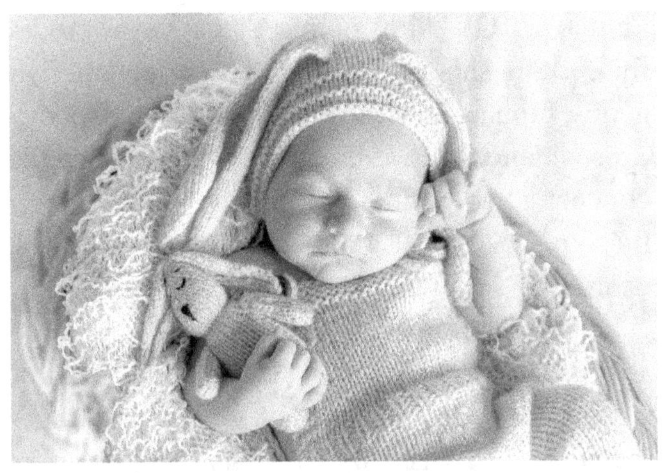

Once upon a time in the vibrant town of Harmonyville, there lived a cheerful baby named Moody. Moody was a bundle of joy with sparkling blue eyes and a contagious giggle that could brighten the gloomiest days. Moody's parents, Emma and James, were overjoyed to have him in their lives.

As Moody began to grow, his curiosity blossomed. She eagerly explored his surroundings, gazing at the world with wonder. One day, as Emma was reading a book about baby sign language, she had a brilliant idea. He decided to introduce Moody to the magical world of communication through signs.

Emma started with simple signs for everyday things. She showed Moody the sign for "milk" by gently tapping her fingertips together. Moody's eyes widened with excitement as he grasped the concept. Soon, he was signing "more" after finishing his meals and "sleep" when he felt drowsy.

The enchanting journey continued as Lily's signing vocabulary expanded. Emma and James introduced signs for animals, colors, and emotions. Lily delighted in signing "dog" when their furry friend Max wagged his tail, and he giggled while singing "happy" when surrounded by loved ones.

One sunny day, Moody and his family decided to visit Harmonyville's lively park. As they strolled along the colorful paths, Moody noticed a group of children playing near the playground. Intrigued, he signed "play" and gestured towards the swings.

To Moody's surprise, the other children understood his signs and happily invited him to join their play. The park echoed with the joyous sounds of laughter and shared communication. Moody's parents beamed with pride as they witnessed the magic of baby sign language fostering connections and understanding among the children.

As Moody continued to explore the world around him, he discovered the power of communication through signing. The town of Harmonyville embraced this delightful method, and soon, baby sign language classes became a cherished community activity.

The tale of Moody's adventures with baby sign language spread far and wide. Families across the town and beyond were inspired to embark on their own journeys of communication with their little ones. Moody's story became a beacon of joy, illustrating the beauty of connection and understanding that baby sign language could bring to families.

And so, in the heart of Harmonyville, the legacy of Moody's magical journey lived on, passed down through generations, as families continued to share the wondrous world of baby sign language with their little ones, creating a community bound together by the universal language of love and signs.

Welcome to the enchanting world of baby sign language, a captivating journey that bridges the communication gap between you and your little one. In this delightful exploration, we embark on a transformative adventure that empowers both parents and infants to engage in meaningful, expressive conversations long before spoken words find their way into the tapestry of communication.

In "Tiny Hands, Big Signs: A Guide to Baby Sign Language," we delve into the heartwarming realm of gestures and symbols, unlocking the extraordinary ability of babies to convey their thoughts, needs, and emotions through the magic of signing. This book is designed as a companion for parents, caregivers, and anyone enchanted by the mesmerizing process of witnessing a baby's first steps into the language of signs.

As we navigate through the pages, you'll discover the science behind baby sign language, unveiling the profound impact it has on cognitive development, bonding, and early language acquisition. We'll delve into practical techniques, offering a treasure trove of illustrated signs that are both engaging and simple for your little one to grasp. From the basic essentials like "more," "eat," and "sleep," to the more nuanced expressions of feelings and desires, each sign is a key that unlocks a door to your baby's inner world.

Prepare to be enchanted by heartwarming anecdotes and success stories from parents who have embraced the beauty of baby sign language. Learn how these tiny gestures not only foster communication but also create an unbreakable bond between caregivers and their precious ones.

Whether you're a first-time parent or a seasoned caregiver, "Tiny Hands, Big Signs" is your passport to a richer, more fulfilling connection with your baby. Join us on this captivating expedition into the realm of baby sign language, where each sign is a stepping stone toward a world where tiny hands speak volumes, and the language of love knows no bounds.

CHAPTER ONE

What is the sign language used by babies?

All of us teach our infants some rudimentary sign language. These are extremely basic gestures, such as pointing, clapping, and waving "bye-bye" or "no." Our children want to express their needs and desires, but because speech development lags behind cognitive ability, they are unable to do so clearly. Since hand-eye coordination develops before speech, babies naturally communicate through gestures.

Building on this innate mode of communication, baby sign language enables infants and young children to express their wants, ideas, and wishes to us in an efficient manner. Infants can pick up simple signals for everyday things like "eat," "sleep," "more," "milk," "play," and "teddy bear" months before they can speak clearly.

What advantages does baby sign language offer?

Being understood is one of the most basic human needs, and studies have shown that by giving infants a way to communicate before their vocal cords are ready for speech, baby sign language helps ease parental frustration.

Numerous other advantages of newborn sign language, according to research, include quickening verbal development and enhancing cognitive abilities. By lowering frustration and providing enjoyable time for teaching signals to your infant, it also improves the link between child and parent.

Does infant sign language have formal status?
American Sign Language (ASL) keyword signals are used in the Baby Sign and Learn system. The primary distinction between baby sign language

and ASL is the use of spoken language in addition to the signs.

Infants who are acquiring spoken language are supported and enhanced by baby signing, which does not teach them a new language. In fact, if a child's speech or language development is delayed, speech and language therapists frequently advise signing.

When Is the Right Time to Teach Your Infant Sign Language?

It is advised that babies learn sign language between the ages of six and twelve months, as this is when they can comprehend and exchange simple signals. Babies may not always be able to communicate with parents through crying, cooing, or grunting noises. Therefore, it is best to begin teaching kids sign language at a young age. Nonetheless, there is never a bad time to start teaching your child sign language—some experts advise as early as four months old. You can start teaching sign language to your infant as early as six months of age. The earliest movements and signs that infants use will determine when to begin teaching them sign language.

When to start teaching their child sign language is a concern shared by most parents. But keep in mind that each child develops at their own rate, so it's better to start as soon as the youngster expresses interest and is ready to communicate. Watch out for their immature conduct.

According to American Academy of Pediatrics spokesman and Encino, California pediatrician Howard Reinstein, "most babies have the physical dexterity and cognitive ability to learn some form of sign language at about eight months" (1). Thus, at nine months of age, your kid will acquire sign language, even though they will eventually start interacting with everything around them.

How Can a Baby Learn Sign Language?
Start with the more common, simpler words. Teaching your infant sign language isn't a difficult task, though. To teach a baby sign language, you need to be patient and diligent. You might try teaching simple sign languages for gestures like patting and clapping. These are a few examples of pract

Start with simple signals: Start with a few simple signals, such "milk," "eat," "more," and "finished," that are connected to your baby's everyday activities.

Make constant, unambiguous gestures: When signing to your child, make sure they can see your face and hands.

Repetition is used: The most important thing to keep in mind when teaching your kid sign language is to acquaint them with it by using the same sign or symbol over and over again. Establish a time for interaction and make an effort to spend that time each day sitting down with your child. For greater comprehension, you may, for instance, teach signals like "eat," "drink," and "more" during meals.

Say the following aloud: Say the word out loud so your infant can learn to associate it. Saying the word "diaper" while changing your baby's diaper is one way to engage them.

Have patience; if your infant is not taking up cues right away, do not become alarmed. Be patient and make the process enjoyable for your child by giving them hugs and kisses.

Pay attention: While your infant is attempting to sign a message to you, pay attention to them. If you are distracted, you might not see how well your kid is progressing with sign language.

Motivate your child: Encourage your baby to imitate you when they do.

Keep it simple: As your infant develops confidence and proficiency with the signs, start with a small number and progressively add more. Maintaining consistency is essential. If you continue the practice on a regular and consistent basis, your baby's communication will gradually become more organic.

Keep trying: Teaching your infant to sign can be enjoyable and fulfilling, but it might take some time for them to pick up the skill. Persist and continue signing with your child.

When should I begin teaching songs?

Since it differs from student to student, there is no one "best age" to begin singing lessons. To learn to sing, nevertheless, you will need to dedicate time for consistent practice, concentration, and willpower.

When they begin singing lessons, students should be old enough to pay attention in class and obey their teacher's instructions. Between the ages of seven and ten is when most kids are ready for this kind of training. But as the human voice develops throughout life, singing lessons are beneficial for pupils of all ages. The indications listed below will help you determine when your child is prepared to begin singing lessons.

Three indicators your child is prepared to begin singing lessons

These three indicators indicate that your child is prepared to start singing.

Your youngster is inspired to sing. Motivated students make greater academic progress and are more successful in their studies. A child is likely ready to begin learning how to sing if they have an interest in music or if they can be heard singing along to the radio.

For at least thirty minutes, your child can concentrate. The secret to learning to sing is to practice consistently. Your youngster should be able to handle singing classes and maintain a regular practice schedule if they can concentrate on a job or projects for thirty minutes.

Your child can dedicate some time to practicing singing. To learn to sing, students must set aside time for practice every day, if not every week, in addition to voice instruction. In order to effectively manage practice time, parents are crucial. The youngster will have more success adhering to their teacher's instructions if they can follow instructions and respond well to coaching.

SUGGESTIONS FOR BEGINNING SINGING LESSONS

- Look after your voice properly. Singers must be aware of maintaining a strong and healthy voice, much as musicians would with their instrument. Pro tip: Students should refrain from yelling and drink lots of water every day to stay hydrated.
- Before singing, warm up. Warming up vocally is essential before every rehearsal or performance. If students sing loudly without warming up, they risk damaging their voices. Vocal students should warm up and extend their voices just like they would before a football or soccer match.
- Develop your ability to distinguish pitch. The secret to voice lessons is ear training. One way to become a better vocalist and raise your pitch is through interval training. During singing sessions, instructors teach students how to train their ears; it is crucial for pupils to develop this ability.
- Every day, practice singing. Perfectionism is attained with practice. Pupils who practice often make progress far more quickly than those who exercise infrequently. Students who dedicate

time each day to practice will eventually surpass their greatest expectations.

• Master the song and its lyrics before honing the technique. Students can concentrate on their singing style and avoid being sidetracked by trying to recall the song's lyrics and melody if they learn and memorize them. You won't believe how much this will assist!

• Join other pupils in singing. Applying topics gained in courses can be enjoyable and productive when done with other individuals through music-making. Pupils can advance far more quickly than those who practice alone when they sing in a band or group context as well as when they practice alone. Singing with loved ones is a joyful and uplifting activity that might inspire you to get well.

CAN I START SINGING LESSONS TOO LATE?

There's always time to start singing! Students of any age might benefit from singing classes because voice lessons actually have a lot of advantages. Singing can also assist kids develop other academic courses and maintain mental and physical acuity.

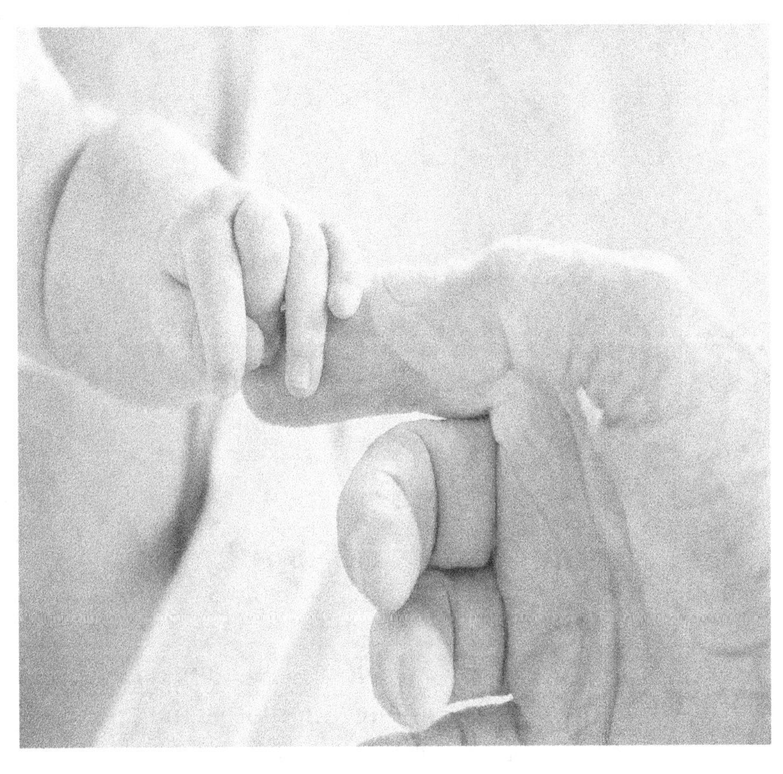

CHAPTER TWO

Fundamentals of Sign Language:

Fundamentals of American Sign Language
Effective ASL communication or signing depends on five factors: handshape, palm orientation, position, movement, and non-manual markers or signals (also known as NMM or NMS). Learning ASL requires an understanding of the criteria since they all impact the meaning and comprehension that is communicated. Let's examine how each option affects some fundamental sign language sentences.

Hand Form

There are more than 55 handshapes available for this parameter, which describes the hand configuration. It's critical to comprehend how handshape relates to fundamental ASL signs because alterations in handshape can have diverse or no meanings. It's comparable to how a single character or sound, like "way" and "why," can alter the meaning of spoken words.

The ASL terms for "school" and "impossible" are comparable examples in basic sign language; they have different hand shapes but the same position, movement, and palm orientation. Thus, the handshapes are what set the words apart from one another.

- Orientation of the Palm

In basic American Sign Language, the palm orientation refers to the position or orientation of the palm. For instance, there are various meanings associated with fundamental sign language words or phrases depending on whether your hand is facing you, down, or upwards. The fundamental sign language terms for "maybe" and "balance," for instance, share the same handshape, placement, and range of motion. In fundamental sign language, the two are distinguished from one another by the palm orientation.

- Whereabouts

The placement of the hand—on your chin, forehead, in the air, on your chest, etc.—is another factor that is crucial to understanding the fundamentals of sign language. The hand's location is more a component of the fundamental words used in sign language than it is a symbol with its own meaning.

For instance, the handshape, movement, and palm orientation of the phrases "apple" and "onion" in basic sign language are identical. The hand's placement—by the temple for "onion" and in the middle of the cheek for "apple"—indicates that the two similar signals have different meanings.

- Motion

An additional component in basic sign language is the way your hands move—up, down, back, forward, diagonally, wave, zigzag, etc. The basic ASL signs for "fly" and "airplane," for instance, are identical in terms of hand form, palm orientation, and placement. But what sets the two apart from one another is the way they move.

Non-Manual Signals and Markers (NMM or NMS)

Non-manual markers or signals, or NMM or NMS, are the final parameter. These are the facial (brows, eyes, nose, lips, and so on), shoulder (lifting), head (nods, tilts, and shakes), and body (tilting) emotions and signals that, when combined with hand gestures, convey meaning. The tone, mood, and intent are represented visually through non-manual signals.

A signer uses all five of these factors for fundamental sign language words within their "space." This space is the region in front of the body, from a few inches above the head to the abdomen or belly button, where the majority of signs are made.

The Most Vital Basic Sign Language Expressions
Acquiring sign language skills requires practice and patience. To get started, you can start by being familiar with some fundamental ASL signs. You can lay the groundwork for future development when you learn the art of sign

language by becoming proficient in a few of the fundamental signals.

We will explain and demonstrate ten fundamental sign language terms for you below. Basic sign language phrases can be taught using written instructions, but the best teachers are the video demonstrations.

Raising your hand with your palm facing out, four fingers held straight and together, and your thumb curled into your palm is how you say "hello" in ASL. To make a salute, bring your four fingertips to your forehead, palm facing out. Then, straighten your hand and arm back to a ninety-degree angle, maintaining the palm orientation and hand form.

What's Up With You?

Two hands are needed to communicate "how are you?" in basic sign language. Make a fist with both hands, palms inside and thumbs facing up, in front of your chest to start. Twist your thumbs in the other direction while bringing your knuckles together at an angle. Once you've twisted the sign to point toward the person you are speaking to, finish it by lifting one hand to indicate an inquiry and raising your eyebrows.

It's good to meet you.
In basic American Sign Language, you would bring your hands up in front of your chest and place the top hand, palm down, on top of the other, palm up (fingers straight and held together, pointing in opposing directions) to say "nice to meet you." The final position should be both hands in fists in front of the shoulders, with the index finger pointing up and the palms facing each other. Next, bring the palms down together in a sliding motion across each other. To complete the sign, bring both hands together until their folded fingers contact, then point with one hand at the individual you are speaking to.

- **What's Your Name?**

In simple sign language, you ask someone their name by putting one hand in front of your chest, pushing forward, facing out, and with your palm facing up. Then, raise both hands in front of the chest, making a fist with the palms facing out and the index and middle fingers pointing straight up.

Bringing both hands together in front of your chest, with fingers pointing outward at a slight angle and one above the other, is how you should hold them. To tap the middle knuckle twice, bring down the top two fingers and tap the bottom two fingers. To close, open your hands with your palms facing up and bring them back together (palms still up!) in front of your chest in two quick waves. This is equivalent to twice moving your open hands side to side while keeping your palms facing up.

- **I Go By...**

As with asking someone their name in sign language, the first step in saying "My name is..." in ASL is to touch your chest with an open hand, palm facing in. Then, once again, make a fist with your index and pointer fingers facing outward at an angle, hitting your middle knuckles twice on each hand. Next, start using the ASL alphabet to spell your name.

- **Many thanks:**

The ASL sign for "thank you" is not too difficult to use. Start with your hand open, thumb held slightly apart, fingers together. To complete the sign, raise your hand back out in front of your face and drop it after momentarily touching your chin with the tips of your four fingers, palm facing inward.

- **Hearing-impaired**

In simple sign language, one hand should be raised, fingers fisted, index finger pointing up, palm facing out, to express "deaf." With the palm still facing out, bring the index finger to your mouth (pointing), then tap your lips. Next, return the index finger in an arc to touch your ear while keeping your hand and palm in the same positions throughout.

- **Observing**

In order to sign "hearing" in ASL, first make a fist with your index finger straight. With the palm of your hand facing inward toward your face, make a pointed finger fist and place it in front of your mouth. With the finger pointing sideways, do an upward and downward circular motion with it in front of your mouth.

- **Hard of Hearing:**

To demonstrate "Hard of hearing" in basic sign language, raise one hand and make a fist, pointing and index fingers straight. Maintain the two fingers pointing away from you and the palm facing sideways. Similar to sketching a rainbow, tap the two fingers once in front of your chest, then slide them up and over in an arcing motion to tap down again.

- **Good-bye**

In ASL, saying farewell is not too difficult. Raise your hand in front of you, fingers and palm facing outward, to start. Bend the top four fingers just at the knuckles three times to bring them down in a waving motion.

Good Resources for Basic Sign Language
It takes practice and time to learn the basics of sign language. Thankfully, there are lots of resources out there to support you and your loved ones on the trip, such as the ones listed below:

Lifewire:
16 Free Resources for Learning Sign Language
Top 10 & 25 American Sign Language Signs for Novices in Smart ASL
Youngs Course: Sign Language for Young People
Children with speech or language impairments can also benefit greatly from a variety of health care resources, such as the in-home speech therapists provided by KidsCare Home Health. Our focus is on providing home health therapy to

children with disabilities, and we are dedicated to providing C.A.R.E. (commitment, accountability, results, and ethics) services to families around the country. Speak with a KidsCare Home Health expert right now.

CHAPTER THREE

Typical Infant Symptoms:

Baby Sign Language: The Top 20 Signs for Babies Using baby sign language before they can speak is a great tool. Teach it to your infant with our comprehensive tutorial, which includes a visual cheat sheet.

How many times have you wanted to just ask your weeping infant to explain what's wrong? We have all the details you need to start communicating with your baby before they speak, including how to use baby sign language.

How to Instruct Your Child in It

1. Commence with the well-known
What kinds of things and activities does a baby typically witness or engage in? There, begin. In order to ensure that you have plenty of opportunity to utilize signs like "more," "milk," "mom," or "dad," start by teaching signs that babies will use regularly.

2. Keep repeating till you reach the end.
The secret is to repeat. Even though it doesn't appear like a newborn is catching up on it, repeat those first few signs frequently. If the baby isn't responding to the first signs you present, you might be tempted to try another sign, but it's crucial to stick to the fundamentals. A baby's vocabulary can be increased by adding additional 4-5 signs to the rotation once they have mastered the first 4-5.

3. Remain composed.
It's a gradual process, so don't expect your child to master it right away. Have fun and give the infant encouragement. When the infant understands and/or imitates your behaviors, give them praise. Make sure the infant can see your hands and maintain a happy expression on your face.

Flash Cards in Baby Sign Language
You'll naturally use these words frequently because they're incredibly pertinent to a baby's daily routine. Recall that repetition is essential.

Additional Baby Sign Language Card - Mama Naturally
Press your fingers against your thumbs while maintaining a straight grip. Next, with your thumbs facing your body, alternately open and close your hands. It resembles making the mouth of an alligator, but on its side.

Mama Natural's "Eat Baby Sign Language" eating card
Turn your fingers to face the sky and tap them repeatedly against your lips using the same handshape as the "more" sign.

Mama Natural's Hungry Baby Sign Language Hungry Card
Slide your palm down to your abdomen, beneath your chin, and press it flat against your chest. Imagine your hand traveling the route that food travels.

- **Milk**

Mama Natural's baby sign language milk card
The sign for "milk" should be familiar to everyone who has ever milked a cow. Consider milking a cow. With your fingers tucked under your thumb and your thumb facing you, make a fist and open and close it like you're milking a cow.

- **Water**

Mama Natural's Baby Sign Language water card
"W" stands for water. Making a "W" with your three middle fingers, putting your thumb and pinkie together out of sight, and tapping your hand against your chin is how you sign for water.

Please use the Mama Natural baby sign language card.
Your kid can be taught to sign "eat," "milk," and "water," after which you can ask them to say "please" before granting their request. All you have to do is place one hand flat against your chest and rotate it in a circle.

Thank You Baby Card in Sign Language - Mama Natural
Give them your gratitude after they've said "please." Make the same gestures as if you were blowing a kiss after tapping your fingertips against your chin.

Mama Natural's "All Done Baby Sign Language" card
With your palms facing you and your fingers spread, raise your hands to your chest. Then flip them out, so the palms face your baby.

Mama Natural's Baby Sign Language Change Card
This symbol is more intricate. Curl both hands' fingers into a ball, excluding the index finger. After tucking it into a hook form, cross your hands at the wrists and alternate them multiple times from top to bottom.

Mama Natural's Potty Baby Sign Language Potty Card
Have you and your child ever played "I've got your nose"? Potty is signed with the same hand shape—thumb tucked between first two fingers. Using your hand, form the shape and shake it back and forth a few times, much to ringing a bell.

Mama Natural's Bath Baby Sign Language bath card

Make both hands into fists and visualize cleaning a baby's back or an old washboard. Rub your torso vertically with your hands.

Mama Natural's "Play Baby Sign Language Play Card"
Man, hang ten. The hand shape—thumbs and pinkies outstretched, other fingers tucked in—became associated with California surfer males for a reason. "Play" is indicated by making the form with both hands and twisting them back and forth at the wrists.

Mama Natural's "Sleep Baby Sign Language Sleep Card"
Start at your forehead with your fingers spread wide and your palm facing you. Next, as you move them down your face, close them. Imagine your eyes closing when you sleep.

Mama Natural's book, Baby Sign Language book card
With your fingers flat and your palms pressed together, open them. Similar to the spine of a book, keep your palms touching at the bottom.

Mama Natural's "Daddy Baby" sign language father's card

Spread your fingers and hold your palm up to make the "daddy" symbol. With your palm pointing sideways, tap your forehead with your thumb.

Mama Natural's Mommy Baby Sign Language Mommy Card
The sole distinction between the signs for "daddy" and "mommy" is that you tap your thumb to your chin instead of using your thumb.

Mama Natural's Dog Baby Sign Language Dog Card
To make the dog sign, place one hand down by your thigh and snap your fingers together, much like you would when you call your dog inside. Use your thumb and middle finger to snap.

Mama Natural's Cat Baby Sign Language Cat Card
The cat symbol is meant to resemble your cat's facial whiskers. Put a hand over your lips in the area where a cat's whiskers grow. Pinch your thumb and index finger together and imagine pulling your hand outwards as if you were running your fingers along the whiskers.

Mama Natural's "I Love You Baby" sign language card
Consider an embrace, which is among the most innate ways to show affection. With your fists balled up like you're embracing yourself, cross your arms in front of your chest.

Mama Natural's "Yes Baby Sign Language Yes Card"
How do we typically say "yes," even when we're speaking? by giving a head nod in both directions. The "yes" symbol simply uses your hand to make the same motion. One hand should be made into a ball and held close to your shoulder. It should then be wagged up and down as though you were nodding "yes."

Assistance
Mama Natural's Baby Sign Language Help Card
How often does your child ask to be hoisted up by reaching out their arms? It's similar to the sign for "help." Put your non-dominant hand's flat palm on top of your dominant hand, which is curled into a thumbs-up position. Position them both below your waist and raise them both up your body such that the lower hand is raising the upper hand.

Chart of Baby Sign Language

Alright, those are the top 20 baby signs in sign language! I've made you and your baby a free one-page printable guide to help you both conquer them!

CHAPTER FOUR

Signs of Mealtime:

Mealtime indicators are essential for creating habits, encouraging dialogue, and improving the dining experience in general. These indicators work as visual cues to help people know when it's time to eat, particularly those who have special dietary requirements or communication difficulties. These signs, which range in complexity from straightforward mealtime symbols to intricate visual schedules, help create an organized atmosphere that is comforting and predictable.

Mealtime signs provide a way for people with cognitive or developmental difficulties to more easily manage their daily routine. Pictures of plates, cutlery, and food items can serve as visual aids to help communicate mealtime expectations. These signs encourage independence by giving people the ability to understand and actively engage in the mealtime ritual.

Mealtime signs are very useful resources in therapeutic and educational contexts. They are used by educators and counselors to make a visual schedule that aids in kids' comprehension of the events that take place during meals. This visual accompaniment facilitates a more seamless transition between activities and helps to lower anxiety.

Mealtime signs can be especially helpful in hospital settings for people recovering from surgery or those with a variety of medical issues. Healthcare practitioners can better explain dietary restrictions, meal times, and necessary preparations when there is clear signage. This promotes the general wellbeing and recuperation of patients in addition to guaranteeing enough nutrition.

The benefits of mealtime signs also extend to families with small children. Mealtimes become more predictable and less stressful for parents and kids when visual cues are used to help toddlers and early children establish a sense of routine. Additionally, teaching kids about various cuisines and table manners may be entertaining and informative with the introduction of mealtime signals.

Essentially, mealtime signals are more than just visual cues; they are forces behind independence, inclusivity, and clear communication. Mealtime signs are a great way to create a supportive and encouraging environment for people of all ages and abilities, whether they are used in homes, schools, hospitals, or other therapeutic settings.

How Can My Baby and I Establish a Mealtime Routine?
Make a special area for your infant if you want to start a mealtime routine with them early on. Your infant will probably have a booster seat or

high chair of their own when they eat at the table. To let your baby know when it's time to eat, get this ready. Some parents enjoy getting their baby involved in meal preparation or cooking. So while you prepare the meal, put your infant in their chair and have a conversation with them. Your baby may feel extra special when they use a certain plate or cup that you provide for them every time. They can also have their own cutlery as they get older.

What Use Does Baby Sign Language Have During Mealtimes?
To help with communication and understanding, it can be a great idea to include some basic sign language into your mealtime routine with your baby. Consider using some baby sign language if you enjoy getting your baby involved in meal preparation. You can communicate that you're preparing food, ask your baby if they'd like a drink and tell them that you're about to put their bib on.

What Are Some Baby Mealtime Signs?

The signs for "food" and "eat" are the same in baby sign language. You might also find the mealtime sign language for bib and drink useful. As your baby gets older, you can progress from drinking and teaching them the different signs for milk and water. In this way, they should be able to communicate to you their preferences, which is all great for their development.

How Do I Know When My Baby is Full?

At mealtimes, it's important to be aware of your baby's fullness cues. If they're pushing away food, turning their head away from the spoon or showing other signs that they are no longer interested in eating then this could mean that they are full. Over time, you will get to know your baby's cues and this will help you understand when it is time for them to stop eating. It's also important to remember that mealtime is a great chance for family bonding and

How Can I Make Mealtimes More Fun?

When it comes to mealtimes, you can make them more fun for your baby by introducing new foods and tastes. Use a variety of textures, flavors, and colors as this will help with their sensory development. Sing songs that are related to food or even put on some music while they eat. You could also try different games such as making funny faces with their food or hide some of their favorite snacks in a bowl of oats and see if they can find them. All these activities will help your baby become more engaged and interested in what they're eating. Finally, always remember to be patient with your baby at mealtimes. They may take longer than you would expect and that's ok! Just keep encouraging them, praising them, and trying to make mealtimes a fun experience.

Step by step Step 1

Mealtime is a meaningful time to introduce sign language to infants. Introduce and review the signs for eat, more, all done, milk, and water during mealtimes. Refer to the Sign Language Cards for help with making the signs (see Resources).

Step 2

Always use the words when you introduce the signs. Infants will likely use the signs first, then use word approximations with the signs, and then eventually the full word. Each child's time frame for this will be different, as children become verbal at different times.

CHAPTER FIVE

Bedtime indicators:

Sleep is essential for overall health, and getting a good night's sleep can be greatly aided by identifying bedtime indicators. This is a thorough approach to recognizing and appreciating these cues for a calm nighttime routine.

1. **Dimming the Lights:** As night falls, your body knows it's time to wind down when the lights are lowered. This aids in controlling melatonin synthesis, the hormone that induces sleep.

2. **Reducing Screen Time**: It's critical to avoid using screens for at least an hour before bed. Electronic device blue light disrupts the creation of melatonin, which makes it more difficult to fall asleep.

3. **Calming Activities**: Before going to bed, partake in peaceful pursuits like light yoga, reading a book, or having a warm bath. Your body receives this signal from these rituals to wind down and be ready for sleep.

4. **Regular Sleep routine**: By creating a regular sleep routine, you can synchronize your body's internal clock. To maintain your circadian rhythm, go to bed and wake up at the same time every day—even on the weekends.

5. **Comfortable Sleep Environment**: Make sure your sleeping environment is in your bedroom. Maintain the space calm, dark, and cold. Purchase cozy pillows and a mattress to improve the quality of your sleep overall.

6. **Mindfulness and Meditation**: Calming a racing mind can be achieved by engaging in mindfulness or meditation exercises before bed. To help you settle into a more peaceful

condition, concentrate on deep breathing or guided relaxation techniques.

7. **Limit Coffee and large Meals**: Steer clear of large meals or caffeinated drinks right before bed. A full stomach and stimulants can interfere with sleep, making it more difficult to get a good night's sleep.

8. **Wind Down Routine**: Create a pre-sleep ritual that alerts your body to the impending night. This could involve taking a warm, caffeine-free beverage, stretching gently, or listening to relaxing music.

9. **Steer Clear of Stimulating Activities**: At least one hour before going to bed, take part in mentally taxing activities like strenuous exercise or contentious conversations. Instead, choose kinder, more peaceful activities.

10. **Understanding Personal Signals**: Be mindful of the distinct cues your body gives you. Your body is preparing for sleep when it yawns, droops its eyes, and naturally loses energy.

You can create the conditions for a more rejuvenating and restful sleep experience by incorporating these bedtime signs into your nightly routine. As you create a space that encourages restful sleep, keep in mind that consistency and mindfulness are key. When you pay attention to the subtle cues that lead you to a restorative night's sleep, sweet dreams are in store.

How Can I Help My Baby Sleep Through the Night?

It can sometimes be easier to go to bed with a baby if you have a routine that you stick to every day. What could be the purpose of adding baby sign language to that routine? These exquisitely illustrated baby sign language posters can help you improve your bedtime communication and assist your baby in understanding that it's time to sleep. You can teach your baby many useful bedtime signs from this helpful collection, such as sleep, bath, and book.

What Are Some Helpful Bedtime Signs For Babies?

As well as helping your baby understand that it's time to go to sleep, bedtime signs for babies can also play a crucial role in teaching your baby what they need to do each day to take care of themselves, such as brushing their teeth or having a good wash in the bath. They can also help you understand why your baby might not be sleeping. They might need their favorite toy or comforter, or they might need a nappy change. Learning these bedtime signs will help improve communication between you and your baby, and hopefully help everyone get some good sleep!

Five Signs Bedtime Should Be Earlier!

- **Hi Lovebugs!**

I find I am always getting the question: what should my baby's bedtime be? Let me tell you, there is no straight forward answer for this. You will find that your baby's bedtime will shift quite often in the first 2 years of life as their sleep needs change, and the number of naps per day changes. Below, I outline the five signs that bedtime should be earlier. If you're curious on what your baby's ideal bedtime and nap times should be, I encourage you to download

Lovebug, take advantage of our free trial, and find out for yourself!

Your baby's bedtime is later than 8pm. Babies, unlike adults, tend to fall asleep in the first few hours of the night (between 5pm and 7pm). If you keep your child up later than 8pm, you could be interfering and even disrupting their natural tendency to fall and stay asleep.

Your baby is waking up in the early morning. I used to think that keeping a baby up later meant they would sleep late into the morning, but after working with tons of families, it's not true. When your baby stays awake past their natural bedtime, they produce adrenaline to keep themselves awake. The adrenaline doesn't wear off quickly, resulting in more wake-ups in the first half of the night and actually causing them to wake EARLIER.

Your baby is fussy, grouchy, or hyper during bedtime routine. Your baby should be calm for the majority of their bedtime routine. If they go into a fussy, grouchy or hyper state, it's usually because they are experiencing a surge of adrenaline.

Your baby had bad naps that day. If your baby is getting less day sleep than we want, they can keep their sleep balance by sleeping at night. If you find your baby had short crummy naps, then an early bedtime will do the trick.

You have a cat nap in the late afternoon. A lot of times, we offer our babies a cat nap in the late afternoon, thinking they just want a nap, but really they are ready to go down for the night. If you are always offering a nap after 4:30pm, try switching that to a 5-6pm bedtime instead.

If you think it's time to move to an earlier bedtime, try starting your bedtime routine 15 minutes earlier each day. You may find that an earlier bedtime means longer nights, fewer wake ups and that they fall asleep more quickly after you put them in their crib.

How Lovebug will customize to your family to determine your baby's ideal bedtime:

All you have to do is log your baby's sleep, and Lovebug will provide you with a custom sleep schedule that updates hourly! Have a day of crummy naps? Lovebug will suggest an early bedtime! Miss a nap, that's ok too! Lovebug will adjust to your child & their sleep needs.

Choose when you want your little one to wake up in the morning! Lovebug will adjust your naps & bedtime to get you there.

What else Lovebug will do to help your family determine baby's ideal bedtime:

Lovebug will sync with your entire care team! Grandma putting baby down so you can have a date night? Grandma's Love Bug app will notify her when it's time to start the bedtime routine.

CHAPTER SIX

Playtime Indications:

Playtime Signs is a comprehensive and entertaining educational resource created to help kids develop early communication abilities. The curriculum promotes language development in an enjoyable and natural way by introducing and reinforcing a range of crucial indicators through interactive activities and visual aids.

Playtime Signs' integration of sign language as a communication tool is one of its main advantages. This method helps young learners develop their motor skills and coordination in addition to helping them acquire language. Through the program, children may successfully express their wants and desires by learning a variety of regularly used signals.

Playtime Signs is different from other traditional language learning approaches since it is interactive. Children are encouraged to actively participate in the learning process through engaging games and activities, which makes learning fun and dynamic. In addition to grabbing young minds, this practical method helps students retain their sign language abilities.

Moreover, Playtime Signs acknowledges the significance of parental participation in the education of young children. The program gives parents the tools and direction they need to get involved in their child's education. This cooperative method fosters a supportive atmosphere for language development while strengthening the relationship between parents and children.

Playtime Signs' curriculum is carefully planned, keeping in mind the developmental stages of young children. Toddlers' needs and interests are taken into consideration while choosing the signals that are taught, making the learning process interesting and meaningful. The methodical and efficient development of children's abilities is facilitated by the progressive escalation of challenge.

Playtime Signs promotes inclusion by including a variety of representations in its visual resources, in addition to its educational advantages. This fosters a sense of acceptance and togetherness in addition to exposing them to a range of cultural elements.

In conclusion, Playtime Signs is a comprehensive curriculum that develops children's cognitive and physical abilities in addition to giving them useful linguistic skills. Playtime Signs fosters good learning experiences for young children and lays a solid foundation for effective communication through its participatory and inclusive approach.

A complete program called Playtime Signs was created to help parents and caregivers communicate with their newborns and toddlers by using sign language.
With the goal of improving early communication abilities, this program presents important indicators linked to typical play activities.
The advantages of playtime signs

Encourages early communication by allowing infants to voice their wants and needs before they are able to do so verbally.
Promotes interactive conversation and a closer bond between caregivers and children, strengthening the parent-child bond.
Boosts cognitive growth: Learning sign language activates brain circuits, contributing to overall development.
Important Playtime Indicators:

"Play" Sign: Learn to use this sign to signal the start of playtime activities. This could entail making a certain hand motion or clapping hands.

Introduce the "Toy" Sign to assist kids in expressing their want to play with toys. One way to do this is to pretend to hold and play with a toy.

Teach the "More" sign to indicate that you would like to play more or ask for more activities. When playtime is changing, this might be a helpful indication.

Tips for Implementation:

The secret is to be consistent in using signs to reinforce knowledge during playtime.

Repetition: To assist kids in connecting signs to certain behaviors or pursuits, repeat signs on a regular basis.

Positive Reinforcement: Construct a positive relationship between communication and praise and encouragement for kids who use signs successfully.

Engaging Exercises:

Playtime Songs: To make learning more interesting, add signs to well-known children's songs.

Use signs to reinforce meaning in a setting that the child is acquainted with during interactive play sessions.

Parental Participation:

Educational Resources: To facilitate learning and application at home, give parents access to resources like workshops, guides, and videos.

Communication Channels: Create channels of communication so that parents may ask questions, discuss their experiences, and get advice on how to use Playtime Signs in a productive way.

Tracking Development:

Observation: To determine a child's level of understanding, watch how they react to signs when they are playing.

Adjustment: Depending on each student's needs and development, change the way you teach or add additional signs.

In summary:

Playtime Signs is a great way to facilitate early communication and create a happy, engaging atmosphere for kids and parents alike.

Caregivers can actively support their children's language development and general well-being by including signs into their playtime routines.

CHAPTER SEVEN

Feelings & Emotions:

Feelings and emotions play a crucial role in how we perceive the world, interact with others, and maintain our general well-being. Emotions, which have their roots in the intricate interactions between neurobiology, psychology, and society, are a potent lens through which we view the world.

Emotions are fundamentally innate reactions to external stimuli that are ingrained in our evolutionary biology as survival-adaptive systems. Emotions such as fear, joy, rage, and sadness weave a vibrant tapestry that shapes our everyday existence. Every emotion has a distinct mark that affects our attitudes, actions, and even bodily functions.

On the other hand, feelings are the cognizant experiences that result from emotions. These are the labels and subjective interpretations we give to the emotional responses-induced changes in cognition and physiology. Essentially, sentiments give our emotional experiences a narrative structure that enables us to express and convey the complexities of our inner states.

Human emotions are complex and wide-ranging, with both positive and negative aspects. Love, joy, and excitement are regarded as positive feelings that promote fulfillment and connection. On the other hand, while grief, anger, and fear can be difficult to deal with, they are essential for warning us about possible dangers, inspiring change, and promoting personal development.

The study of emotions takes into account societal and cultural factors in addition to personal experiences. Social norms and cultural expectations impact how people interpret and express their emotions, which in turn affects how they negotiate relationships and social institutions. When negotiating the intricacies of social interactions, emotional intelligence—the capacity to identify, comprehend, and regulate one's own emotions as well as those of others—becomes essential.

Emotions and sentiments are important when it comes to mental wellness. Disturbances in the regulation and expression of emotions are frequently observed in conditions like trauma, anxiety, and depression. In order to encourage healing and resilience, therapeutic treatments frequently involve investigating and comprehending these emotional patterns.

The rich complexities of emotions can be powerfully expressed and explored via the genres of art, literature, and music. In addition to fostering empathy and understanding across a range of emotional experiences, they offer a forum for people to connect with and reflect on their own emotional landscapes.

What is it—an emotion or a feeling?

We've all seen paintings of old west bar fights. Someone will snap when something is written or said. I'm not kidding. Hatred, rage, or both simultaneously. When two individuals argue, it's possible that their strong feelings are resolved through communication, or it's not (online interactions tend to fall into the latter category).

A flame war ensues as a result of the furious people inviting allies to express (and defend) their strong feelings. If this outburst is not handled, people learn that it's acceptable to let their emotions run wild and the behavior continues uncontrolled. Even if reasonable people may make an effort to deal with the emotional problems, emotional awareness fades when alliances are formed and people begin to discuss their feelings in public. At that point, emotional decisions cease to be decisions at all and start to seem justified.

In my book, The Language of Emotions, I refer to strong emotions like anger and hatred—as well as panic and the desire to commit suicide—as "raging rapids emotions" because, without understanding their intended purpose or the gifts they hold, it's easy to get swept away by them, pulled under, and repeatedly slammed against the rocks! Instead of being their partner, you could turn into a puppet of your own feelings.

The first step in managing strong, intense, or unsettling emotional states is realizing that while feelings are always true (about something), they aren't necessarily accurate.

Emotions are the primary source of information about everything in your environment; without them, it is impossible to reason, think, learn, make decisions, or communicate. When your emotions are particularly strong, though, you should interject cognitively controlled breaks between experiencing, feeling, and expressing them.

When it comes to anger and hatred, you need to take very long cognitive pauses because if you don't recognize that you're feeling these emotions in the first place, or if you use them inappropriately, you could really harm both yourself and other people.

However, in order to make those essential cognitive pauses, you must first comprehend the distinction between an emotion and a feeling.

What distinguishes emotions from feelings?

Last year, I was asked to explain the distinction between an emotion and a feeling, and I said that an emotion is a noun and a feeling is a verb. I've given the distinction a lot of attention, but I never really understood why it was significant. I was genuinely perplexed as to why there was so much uncertainty - after all, you feel and identify an emotion, right? Correct?

Then, you know exactly how to deal with it since you are aware of the type of feeling it is. Correct? Why, it's so easy that a kid could...

Thud.

I understand that many people find it more difficult.

I went back to the books and eventually understood what was going on after reading

Antonio Damasio's books again (Descartes' Error, The Feeling of What Happens, and Looking for Spinoza), as well as some books on the sociology and neurology of emotion (How Emotions Work by Jack Katz, The Emotional Brain by Joseph LeDoux, and On Being Certain by Robert Burton).

It is the distinction between possessing and being aware.
A feeling is your conscious awareness of the emotion itself, whereas an emotion is a physiological experience (or state of consciousness) that provides you with information about the outside environment. Since I don't really see a significant difference between feeling and emotion, I hadn't really understood why the distinction was so important. I mean, I feel everything that's going on emotionally. Bing.

However, this isn't always the case.

To be honest, a lot of individuals don't even realize they are feeling anything. For them, there is little connection between the emotion and the consciousness of it; they are not even aware that they are afraid, furious, or unhappy. It takes a strong emotional condition to push them into a severe mood (or for someone else to notice it) before they can recognize that they have been feeling particularly depressed, anxious about money, or furious at work.

Many people have no awareness of their emotions at all, or there is a gap between their feeling and their emotions. They are unaware that they are feeling this way. They aren't feeling it clearly, but the emotion is undoubtedly present and is shown (at least to others) via their actions.

Perhaps they require a chart to illustrate the various feelings! We are grateful that the Department of Lolcats has given us one!

A picture of a cat's feelings

But honestly, I speculate in my book that this mismatch between feelings and emotions results from the anti-emotional conditioning we receive—emotions are taught to be the antithesis of spirituality, the antithesis of reason, and the source of all human problems—and that this misperception is wrong [ish].

People have, in my opinion, been socialized from birth to suppress, repress, ignore, demonize, and avoid their emotions, which is why I believe they are unaware of them. Alternatively, they go to the other extreme and let their feelings flare up right away.

Nobody is benefiting from this instruction. Because an unfelt emotion can twitch around inside of us like an overactive pinball, it causes us to become emotionally oblivious as well as emotionally chaotic.

Fortunately, you can become more conscious and knowledgeable about your emotions if you are able to feel them. Additionally, feeling and understanding your emotions can really help you deal with them, despite the horrible training we receive about them.

Being able to name, feel, and know
According to intriguing research on emotion recognition by UCLA's Mathew Lieberman, you may seemingly relax your brain and yourself just by naming an uncomfortable emotion. According to Lieberman's research, there is a positive correlation between experiencing emotions,

having feelings, and being able to cognitively identify emotions.

In my book, I discuss how to use your linguistic and cognitive skills to recognize, express, and validate your feelings. Based on my decades of experience as a practitioner and educator, I have found that doing so accomplishes three goals:

1) It aids in the development of emotional awareness and identification, which promotes self-control and concentration;

2) It makes you more emotionally aware by assisting you in comprehending the how, why, and when your emotions occur;

3) It uses your language abilities to assist and communicate with the feeling so you may draw lessons from it and respond in a healthy, sensitive way.

It's a big step from the stale, old "emotions are the opposite of rationality" nonsense to use your language intelligence to support your emotional awareness as taught in The Language of Emotions.

Emotions are by no means the antithesis of reason. Emotions are body language reflecting your environment. Emotions are just data, and you are the one who interprets them. The way you work with and understand your emotions will determine whether or not the result is logical.

The state of neuroscience today demonstrates the critical role that emotions play in our ability to think and make decisions. Emotions and reason can work together as allies rather than as enemies if we can develop the ability to feel emotions rationally.

Emotions need to be felt, named, and understood; this is especially true when they are strong, uneasy, or dangerous.

Flow diagrams!
Let's examine the most straightforward, healthful route from feeling to action (these flowcharts are obviously oversimplified, and there is a lot more complexity involved, but these general concepts are important to grasp):

Feeling → Emotion → Naming → Taking Action based on the information the emotion gives

Let's include melancholy in this flowchart. This would be the process: I feel an emotion, which I believe to be sadness; I name the sadness; and I undertake whatever action my sadness demands (which could include, but are not limited to, sighing, slowing down, releasing tension, or sobbing).

But hold on! Let's not overlook the circumstances and stimuli that cause emotions; I did not include them. Anything that makes you feel something, even your own ideas, might be considered an emotional circumstance. Emotions alert you to potential problems, which may involve your own ideas.

Take note of the word "evoke" that I've used here. Emotions have developed over millions of years to help you comprehend and react to the world; they are not something that just appears in your head or that you think. Your body and mind contain emotions, which are triggered by particular circumstances.

An emotionally charged scenario → Feeling → Emotion → Naming → Taking action based on the information the emotion gives

But hold on once more! You can be seeing things incorrectly!

For example, you might be afraid of a coiled rope just like you would of a snake. Alternatively, you may experience reality incorrectly if your beliefs arouse your emotion. If you don't regularly pause to reflect on your thoughts, they may not be correct. You could make a poor or harmful decision if you act on an emotion that was aroused by unfounded situations.

Even when a situation has nothing to do with emotion, it might nevertheless arouse feelings. Your body may react as though there is a frightening stimulus present, for example, if your heart rate or adrenaline level increase.

Similarly, your body may react as though you are happy or angry whether you are frowning or smiling. For example, it may be that you are frowning and slouching without realizing it, and this is triggering your anger and melancholy! Emotions provide you with important information about something that is happening, but it is up to you to identify what it might be.

That's why I included a step that should help you recognize the issue and (hopefully) determine what's actually going on.

An emotionally charged scenario → Emotion → Feeling → Naming → Engaging with the emotion → Taking action based on the knowledge the emotion offers OR opting out of action since the situation doesn't call for it

I realize this looks like a long journey, but if you have your emotional talents down, you can finish it in a flash. It's not challenging.

Ultimately, it's considerably more difficult to aimlessly navigate life, subjected to feelings you are unable to recognize or comprehend.

Let's examine fury.
So let's add anger to the flowchart and examine how it functions when individuals decide to lose their cool.

Your identity, perspective, or voice are threatened. → You become angry. → You don't take the time to identify your anger; instead, you heap insults and assumptions upon it. → You become even more angry. → You attack. → The other person retreats or retaliates. → Rinse and Repeat. → Welcome to Hell.

Ah, that flowchart, we all know it! It is active virtually every day on the internet and in Congress and the U.S. Senate!

Let's take another look at rage, this time with cognitively controlled pauses (notice that neither of these flowcharts describes a rage disorder, which is characterized by circumstances that are frequently linked to untreated depression, other neurochemical variables, or possibly PTSD).

Anger is evoked when something threatens your voice, viewpoint, or sense of self. You feel the anger, name it, and note how intense it is. This gives you a moment to gather yourself and ask yourself the questions that anger evokes: What do I value? What needs to be protected and restored? You identify the problem, establish boundaries without resorting to violence, and restore your sense of self without violating the humanity of the other person. Congratulations! Your anger has been resolved.

Did you note that in the second flowchart, there was no need to become angry? You don't have to jump into the roaring rapids every time an emotion shows up if you know that you're experiencing it, that you can recognize it, and that there are particular actions you can do to look into the matter.

No matter what is happening to you or around you, having emotional skills gives you options, freedom, and breathing room.

Thus, an emotion provides you with knowledge about a situation that is emotionally significant. It provides you with an account of your perceptions and experiences.
As the partner of your emotions, it is your responsibility to experience the emotion, identify it, pose the right questions, and behave in a way that is both sensible and feeling. I'm arguing that it's feasible, in addition to being essential for the wellbeing of your relationships, your community, and your mental health.

Why, it's so easy that a kid could do it

Well, I won't go that far, but once you get the hang of it, learning how to feel your emotions becomes simple, enjoyable, and illuminating!

More significantly, you and your huge, intense, potentially hazardous emotions will become less toxic when you learn to recognize, name, and take the required, cognitively-moderated breaks to help you determine whether the scenario (or your reaction) is legitimate.

assistance with your emotional and naming abilities
Here on my website (and on Facebook), we used compassionate community sourcing to build our Emotional Vocabulary List. All the emotions have been categorized (angers, fears, etc.) and intensified (soft, medium, and intense) by me and my empathic group.

For example, there are terms for mild, medium, and severe rage in this list; anger does not exist on its own. For despair, fear, guilt, happiness, and so forth, we have taken the same actions.

As they share their newfound emotional awareness with the people in their lives, readers of The Language of Emotions have asked for this list. We made this list to help people become aware of different emotional intensities and to develop better emotional articulation and awareness. According to reports from my empathic comrades, many people lack a functional vocabulary for their emotions because they are lacking in the feeling and naming areas from the flowchart above.

As UCLA's Matthew Lieberman found, you can manage and even calm your emotions just by naming them. Having a specific emotional vocabulary is essential for emotional skill and empathic awareness, and our list can help you with that. Please feel free to forward this list to your loved ones!

In summary, feelings and emotions are essential aspects of the human experience that permeate all aspect of our life. Comprehending and accepting the intricacy of our emotional existence not only improves our self-awareness but also cultivates deeper relationships with others. We go on a deep journey of self-discovery and interpersonal understanding as we negotiate the ups and downs of emotions, weaving more nuance and significance into the fabric of our common human experience.

CHAPTER EIGHT

Daily Tasks:

A view of a woman packing groceries into her car from the back.

You might become even more active if you reconsider what you consider to be exercise.

Getty Images / Mypurgatoryyears

Although most people are aware of the health advantages of exercising, the Centers for Disease Control and Prevention report that less than 25% of US adults meet weekly exercise guidelines. Therefore, it's likely that you struggle to find the motivation to work out even though you know it's important for everyone to do so on a regular basis.

What then goes wrong?

People don't exercise more for a variety of reasons. It's possible that you lack the tools you believe you need, or you're pressed for time or energy.

When you think of "exercise," however, you might picture sneakers, sports bras, and weight benches. However, you don't need to work out at a gym to meet the CDC's recommendations for physical activity. Actually, the word "exercise" appears not once in the 23% number included in the CDC's 2018 National Health Statistics report. Rather, the focus is mostly on mobility and physical exercise, whether for leisure, job, or medical reasons.

Physical exertion was a part of everyday life for most of human history in the form of work and housework. People spend a lot more time sitting still these days—on couches, in desk seats, and in their cars. However, physical activity is still necessary for a healthy lifestyle, and it may be simpler to reach your daily exercise goals by doing things you must do (like mow the grass) rather than making time for a dedicated workout.

You might be motivated to become even more active if you reevaluate what you consider to be exercise. If you choose to sweep instead of go to the gym, you're not necessarily losing out. This is important to know.

A person with a skateboard and paper bag walks a bulldog.
The effects of informal exercise are equivalent to those of structured workouts.

supersizer via Getty Pictures

Do routine tasks truly qualify as exercise?

In a nutshell, sure. Expert and world-class powerlifter Robert S. Herbst says, "Your body can't tell the difference between bending down to pick up a kettlebell and bending over to pull out a weed."

Formal and casual exercise are the two categories into which experts classify exercise. As the owner and head physiotherapist of Ireland's RAPID clinic, Mike Murphy asserts that most individuals do not consider informal exercise to be true exercise. This could be the case because it's hard to measure informal exercise; walking for an hour appears easier to measure than doing housework. However, Murphy pointed out that a lot of daily duties actually consume a lot more energy than modest exercise.

"Everyday walking up and down stairs, to the shops, carrying things, hanging clothes out to dry, etc. -- all of these activities build up and over weeks and months these can significantly influence our energy balance (contributing significantly to weight gain or weight loss)," he said.

As Nike master trainer and performance coach Brian Nunez put it, some structured workouts even purposefully imitate the "primal movement patterns that represent our daily movement patterns for life," like squatting, pushing, pulling, and twisting. We refer to these courses as "functional training." Conversely, a fitness routine that consists of non-exercise activity thermogenesis, or NEAT exercise, as opposed to structured exercise.

In summary, don't minimize the physical activities you partake in even if you don't plan to work out. Activities that don't need physical activity are a fantastic way to enhance your health, make duties easier, and lower your chance of injury (no more straining a muscle when carrying the groceries in).

These ten commonplace activities qualify as exercise, per experts.

A young man sweeping leaves on the deck has a prosthetic limb.
One of the best ways to accomplish chores and get exercise is to clean the house.
Johnny Greig/Thinkstock

lawn or yard maintenance
It's a real workout, as anyone who has ever mowed the grass by hand in the sweltering heat knows. According to Nunez: "Aside from the low impact and cardiovascular benefits, mowing the lawn requires a lot of functional movement primal patterns in the process of setup, mowing the lawn and cleanup."

Other yard tasks that provide an excellent workout include wedding, gardening, leaf or snow shoveling, and many more.

- **executing errands**

Who says you can't stroll around Target's aisles for your regular hour-long walk? But really, running errands frequently requires a lot of walking, hauling, lifting, and other physical labor.

- **tidying the home**

Moving furniture around the house, climbing and descending stairs, pushing and pulling a mop or broom, and other physical tasks can all be part of cleaning.

- **Taking the dog for a stroll**

Do we really need to say more? While you may be more focused on making sure your dog gets enough exercise on their daily walk, remember that you are also getting your steps in during that time.

Older woman strolls along a street bordered with trees with a little, fluffy puppy.
A stroll around the block will help you meet your daily step goal.
Maskot and Getty Images
Anywhere, one can walk
It's possible that you've heard that prolonged sitting is unhealthy. However, it's beneficial to get up and move around every thirty minutes or so. Walking is also a terrific kind of exercise, whether you're just going to the mailbox, greeting a coworker down the hall, or obtaining a snack.

'I'm running late' sprint
Just to get to the bus or train during the day is definitely a significant amount of light- to moderate-intensity exercise if you use public transit frequently. Furthermore, there's extra work involved if you have to jog a little since you're running late.

- **Having fun with children**

Do you have children in your life? You will run out of breath quite fast if you sit on the nearest couch or bench and watch them play instead of participating in it.

- **Dancing**

You may be the kind who prefers "solo dance party in your pajamas" or perhaps you enjoy going out to dance. In any case, be aware that dancing can provide an excellent cardio and full-body workout.

In a large house, a young woman dances with a small infant.
Dancing is a very aerobic, full-body workout.
Spanish-language/Getty Images
giggling
Do you know what "laughter yoga" is? A 2014 study discovered that laughter yoga works the abs more effectively than exercises like crunches or back lifts. Thus, it is great if you can discover humor throughout your day.

Engaging in sexual activity
Another moderate-intensity workout is having sex. Even more energy is expended than with weight training, however this obviously depends on the particular exercise.

Learn which vitamins to consume and how to determine your health without the use of tests or equipment for further tips on staying in shape outside of the gym.

- **Increased exercise**

Five Elements That Affect How Fast You Gain Muscle

The Method for Almost Free Gym Membership Acquisition

The Greatest Action You Can Take Now to Improve Your

- **Health:**
- **Getting Up**

This article's content is not meant to be used as medical or health advice; rather, it is solely meant to be educational and informative. Any queries you may have concerning a medical issue or your goals for your health should always be directed toward a doctor or other trained health expert.

Common Questions and Answers
Index

Quick Reference for Baby Sign Language Book
Acknowledgments

Gratitude and Special Mentions
About the Author

Author's Journey and Commitment for Baby Sign
Language Book
Note: Always consult with a healthcare
professional or before making significant
changes to Baby Sign Language Book,especially
For Babies

BY
[HUNTER MOODY]

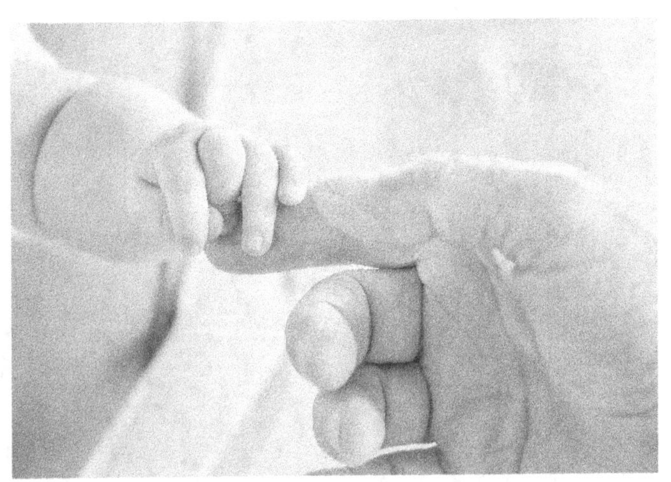